How to Stop Premature Ejaculation:

Proven Method to Enjoy a Bigger, Stronger Penis and Last Longer in Bed Almost No One Knows

Copyright

Disclaimer

This information is not presented by a medical practitioner and is for educational and informational purposes only. The content is not intended to be a substitute for professional medical advice, diagnosis, or treatment. Always seek the advice of your physician or other qualified health provider with any questions you may have regarding a medical condition. Never disregard professional medical advice or delay in seeking it because of something you have read.

Contents

Copyright _____ 2

Disclaimer _____ 3

Introduction _____ 7

Chapter 1 - Your Size _____ **11**
   Measurements _____ 13
   Soft Measurement _____ 13
   Hard Measurement _____ 14
   Thick Measurement _____ 15
   Getting Bigger _____ 16
   Increasing Length _____ 18
   Pull and Slap _____ 19
   The Twirl _____ 20

Chapter 2 - Understanding Your Body _____ **21**
   Excitement _____ 21
   Plateau _____ 22
   Orgasm _____ 22
   Resolution _____ 23
   Your Arousal Patterns _____ 24
   Stage 1 _____ 25
   Stage 2 _____ 26
   Stage 3 _____ 26
   Stage 4 _____ 27
   Your PC Muscles _____ 29

Chapter 3 - Premature Ejaculation _____ **31**
   Functions and Causes _____ 32
   Genetics _____ 34
   Stress and Anxiety _____ 35
   An Unhealthy Lifestyle _____ 36
   Poor Masturbation Methods _____ 37
   The Wrong Posturing _____ 37
   How to Cure Yourself _____ 38
   Premature Ejaculation Myths _____ 39
   Lack of Sexual Experience _____ 40
   Porn Actors Have it Easy _____ 41

You Have Issues _____ 41
Distractions _____ 42
It's Not the End _____ 43

Chapter 4 - Being Healthy and Safe_____**45**
Necessary Nutrients _____ 46
Safety Tips _____ 47
Lubricant _____ 48

Chapter 5 - Exercises _____**51**
Warm-Ups _____ 52
A Warm Shower _____ 53
Hot Wraps _____ 53
Passing Your Limits_____ 54
The Jelqing Technique_____ 54
The Natural Technique _____ 56
Cooling Down _____ 56

Chapter 6 - Improving Your Skills_____**59**
Making Sure Your Partner is Relaxed _____ 59
The Practice Round _____ 60
Using a Condom _____ 61
Distractions _____ 62
Positioning_____ 63
Her Sensitive Areas _____ 64
The Ears_____ 65
The Spine_____ 65
The Neck _____ 66
Oral Sex _____ 67
It's Not About You _____ 69
The Aftermath _____ 70

Conclusion _____**71**

Introduction

Unfortunately, the issue of being unable to last for a long time in bed has been deemed quite problematic for men of all ages.

In addition to that, a man's issue in bed also affects his partner. Women would want their man to last long enough to give them an orgasm and, if he can't, then both the couple's sex lives will be at risk.

There are a few reasons as to why bedtime might not sound so great as it did back then. Obviously, one of the main reason that we will discuss in this book will be premature ejaculations, which is the process of when a man reaches his peaking point too quickly for his partner to feel much of anything during sex.

Another reason would be your sex skills. How good are you in bed? Rather, how good do you think you are? Unfortunately, the basic inserting and thrusting isn't going to do you much good if you want to last for a long time.

In addition, how are you letting your partner feel you? Are you at the right size where your partner can feel you inside of them or are you blankly thrusting in them?

There are other options available to you that you have probably heard of already but never bothered implementing. It's even better if you've never heard them at all since you'll be able to use them as soon as you finish reading. You'll be a lot more enthusiastic in trying out a new method rather than something that you've heard before.

Truthfully, this book will save you a lot of time. That's why you're reading it in the first place. Nowadays, when you want to find an answer to your problems you can simply search up the answer online.

Unfortunately, since there are many options that you can choose from, you aren't sure of which to pick first. Also, in the case where you've picked the wrong site with the information that you don't want, you'd be wasting your time reading through what you already know.

Granted, you probably already know a few things mentioned in this book, but at least your information will be all in one chunk rather than multiple webpages online. Nevertheless, you should read everything seriously and precisely.

You won't know whether you might learn something new if you don't bother relearning at all. It's always good to review on what you know in case if you had missed something earlier on, which might also be one reason for your current problems.

A good advice for you to remember is to not rush. This book might give you the facts and methods that you wanted to know, but it does not mean that you're going to get it immediately.

All results is built upon time and effort and that's the only way you're going to see any improvements. Do not bother stressing yourself out thinking that by skimming for the easiest and quickest method will guarantee you immediate results.

Note that any changes made to your body will always take time to adjust and altered. Since this part of your body is more sensitive than certain areas, you need to expect a longer waiting time for the best results.

Give your body at least two months to start the change. The wait will be worth it and giving up half way isn't going to get you any closer to your desired goal.

Also, don't worry. This book will be giving you natural methods that you can do that don't require you to undergo any type of medication. Although it may take a little more time, it's a lot faster and you're guarantee a lasting result.

Chapter 1 - Your Size

First, before we head off towards any additional facts, dos and don'ts, safety procedures, and skill improvement techniques. We need to first look at the current situation, meaning that you have to look at what you lack and what you want.

You can't expect to continue on with the program if you don't know what your main problem is in the first place. Even if we're going to go through it all, it'll be a lot easier for you to know which piece of information it is that you want to take in during your improvement stage. Besides, your issues now will determine how your results will be in the future.

So, starting off, you need to measure your penis size. You're going to have to measure it as a starting point so bust out a ruler, a notepad, a writing utility, and start measuring. This might even sound like a fun activity for most men out there.

Surely, there is a certain time in a man's age where he will brag about his size to his friends. Normally, it happens more often during the growing stage than any other time period. Young men tend to see it as a competition as to who has the bigger size. Therefore, it's not something that should embarrass you while you're doing it.

Secondly, you'll be focusing on how to make your current size bigger than it is now. Note that you should be realistic about this.

For some men, size is a big problem for a successful sex life. However, after measuring yourself, if you know that you're big then don't bother going through exercises that will make it bigger.

There's a certain limit for all sizes so don't waste your time improving a size that's not going to change. So, for those of you who can change your size, take a moment to think about how big you can get at the end of this book and strive for it.

In addition, we'll also be focusing on helping you get the size that you want. This section will also include tips on how to make you look bigger than what you normally were.

Lastly, we'll be focusing on increasing your length of your penis. Remember, bigger doesn't mean better. You always want to take your partner's size into consideration. Whether you'll be doing the basic front style or doggie style, it doesn't matter.

Even if those two parts of a woman's body can stretch, it doesn't mean that you can't potentially hurt her. The point of sex is to make her feel good at all times, not give her pain when you try to thrust into her.

Measurements

So the key to improvement is to first know what to improve on. Always have a starting point so you can make an ending point.

So first thing's first, you need to pull out a ruler and a measuring tape. You do want to make note of what your size is after each measurement to know what your standing point is at.

Unless if you're not embarrassed by anyone else knowing about your complex, you do want to put that information in a place where only you would know. The reason why trying to remember your size isn't recommended is because you can forget or mistaken the measurement at a later point in time. Basically, you want to be accurate and taking notes is always mistake free.

There are actually three different types of measurements that you have to do with your penis. It's not just about the length but also the width that's important. Make sure that you do take this first step seriously. Although it may seem easy, it can become a real hassle later on if you were to make a careless mistake.

Soft Measurement

This should be the first measurement that you start with simply because it's the most convenient. Soft measurement is basically when you measure your penis when it is still soft, or flaccid.

This is also the most important measurement that you will be focusing on throughout your improvement stages because this is where your progress still start showing up before any other.

In order do your soft measurement you have to make sure that your penis is parallel to the floor. From there, grab your ruler, press it against your pubic bone, and measure to the tip of your penis. Make sure that the measurement is as accurate as possible. If you round make sure that you do not round the numbers up too much.

Hard Measurement

Your hard measurement is the measurement of when you are erected, or when you're hard. It can be challenging to do this type of measurement since mistakes are always possible. However, if you know what you're doing then you will be fine.

When starting, make sure that you are erect obviously. It doesn't matter how you get there just as long as you can keep it there until you're done with your measurement.

Make sure that your erection is at its best when you're doing this measurement because that's where the best results will come out. Just like how you did your soft measurement, you're going to do the same with your hard measurement.

Grab it, make it parallel to the floor, press the ruler against your pubic bone, and measure to the tip of the head of your penis. If you don't like using this method to measure your erection then there are also other ways of doing it.

However, that's something that you have to figure and experiment on your own. Try changing the angle of measurement to see if you are getting the same results as the first one. If you are then stick with whichever angle that you feel most comfortable with.

Thick Measurement

Finally, this is our last measurement: the thick measurement. In this measurement, you will be measure the thickness of your erect penis. You want to use some sort of measuring tape to do this.

Make sure that it's soft and won't hurt you in any way. If you don't have a measuring tape then use some sort of string that you can measure with. As long as you're able to keep track of what your measurements are then any thing will do really.

Thick measurement is very easy to do. Make sure that your erection is still as perfect as possible when you do this. Otherwise, your results won't be as accurate.

Simply take the measuring utility and wrap it around the middle of your penis. If you're using a string then simply mark down where the length stopped and measure it again with a ruler for a more accurate reading.

Getting Bigger

Now that you've gotten your measurements done, we'll be focusing on how to make you get bigger than the size that you are at now. In order to do that, you need to know a little bit about your body.

Here it the quickest and simplest body breakdown that you will ever see: Your penis has three chambers that absorbs the flow of blood, causing an erection.

If you can expand these three chambers, your penis will indefinitely grow bigger than before. Keep in mind that if your thick measurement is already too big then your overall measurement isn't going to improve as much as you want it to.

There are a few simple tips as to how you can make your penis grow bigger. One way is to cut your pubic hair. Now that may seem like a lot of work but it really does help in making you seem bigger than before.

In fact, your pubic hair does take up a good portion of your actual size. Try shaving it and you'll be able to see the difference in size immediately.

Although it doesn't actually change your size, it'll give you the overall look, which should be good enough as to what you're trying to accomplish so far. Besides, shaving your pubic hair will also be good for you later on.

It'll make you feel a lot cleaner and it'll help make your later exercises easier to do without having to withstand the pain of having to pull out hair in the process.

Another tip is to lose weight. It's going to be hard and it's going to take work, but if you want results than you have to work hard for it. Now some people actually believe that big people tend to have a big penis.

Truthfully, that's not the case. In fact, that's not even a proper answer. If you're overweight, you have to pay attention to this. If you're not then keep this in mind: if you are overweight, you will be small, ultimately.

If you are unfit you will be at a normal length. If you are fit then you are good where you are and you just have to brush up on some of your bed skills.

Anyhow, you lose one inch in penis length for every thirty-pound that you are overweight. It's a fact because your actual length will ultimately be hidden under your body fat.

Eat healthy and take in proper nutrients for your body. Your immune system needs it, you need it, and your whole body needs it.

You'll not only be healthy but you'll be getting the results that you want. In the end, you'll be killing two birds with one stone. Also, take in fewer amounts of sugar and carbon dioxide, which means less sugary drinks and sodas in your life.

Start drinking more water if you haven't already done so, preferably about 3-4 bottles per day. Try not to go over the bottles per day rule on water. Although water might be good for your body because it cleans off unnecessary acids, it can also kill your body if you have too much in one day.

Lastly, you do want to do a bit of exercising here and there. If you're on a tight schedule then a simple job in the park or a walk around your neighborhood will be fine. Anything that keeps you healthy and active at all times.

Don't try to slack off too much. Try to tone up your body if you can even if you're doing it for looks rather than health benefits. If you haven't realized this by now, your penis isn't a muscle.

It's a tissue. It's not going to get bigger because your body is now toned. It's going to get bigger because of the biological reasons behind it.

Increasing Length

In this section, we'll be focusing on increasing the length of your penis. Remember, bigger doesn't always mean better as length is important too. Fortunately, there are certain methods as to how you can increase your length without having to perform any difficult exercises.

Most of these methods are basic stretching exercises designed for increasing your length. Of course, you still have to be careful not to make a mistake during the workout.

Make sure that you are soft throughout the whole exercise. If you end up feeling an erection coming up then stop and wait until the feeling has passed before starting again.

Pull and Slap

For this method you need to wrap two of your fingers around your penis. Think of it as putting up an OK sign around yourself. Make sure that the rest of your hand is wrapped around your penis the same too.

When you're in this position, make sure that you are holding your penis just below the tip, or the head. Hold it tightly enough so that it your hand won't let go of it during the workout, but not so much that you're putting rough pressure on it.

Once you're in position, stretch your penis forward and hold it for twenty seconds. When stretching, if it begins to hurt then it means that you are stretching it too much. Always stretch a little bit each time.

When you're ready, slap your penis on the left and right side about 15 times each. Once you're done, change angle. It doesn't matter if you start with the left angle or the right as long as you do both at the end of the workout.

When you change the angle of where you're holding your penis, hold it for 20 seconds before doing the slapping section. Make sure that you're slapping both the left and right side despite the angle of where you're holding.

The Twirl

This method requires you to be in the same position as the pull and slap method. The difference is that when you start, you have to pull your penis outward, just in the opposite way as when you masturbate.

Once you're done, start over from the starting position. Repeat this pattern about 10 times before heading off into the next step. After the first step, start twirling your penis clockwise and counterclockwise five times each.

After the first section, start moving your penis to the left and right while repeating those steps. Unlike the pull and slap method, all steps are the same regardless of direction.

Chapter 2 - Understanding Your Body

So before we go more in-depth as to what could possibly wrong with you, whether it's a lack of skill or an issue of premature ejaculation, you must first understand how the lower part of your body works.

The reason is because, by understanding your reaction to sexual stimulation, you are able to better control your ejaculations during sex.

Of course, in order to be able to do that, you need to become aware of different sexual arousal levels. Now, this is an old theory that was invented years ago. However, it is used by many Sex Therapists to explain to their clients how their body works.

Basically, your arousal levels during sex are split up into four stages: excitement, plateau, orgasm, and resolution. These four stages are not hard to understand but it will be good for you to keep in mind when you try to control yourself during sex.

Excitement

The excitement stage is the first stage of your arousal level. This is the most basic stage that every man will go through, which is basically the erection stage.

The reason why men cannot hold their erection for more than six minutes is because Mother Nature had made it so that men will reproduce as quickly as possible. Thus, that semen has to come out as quickly as they form. It will only take a couple of minutes for an erection to fully form and a few more minutes for it to die down.

Plateau

During this second stage, it is possible that your erection is starting to reach its peak before you have the urge to let it all go. Once this happens, you will start to realize that your breathing rate and heart rate are increasing.

Also, during this stage, you will also experience what is known as pre-cum. Basically what that is, is when there is a slight discharge from the penis. Although it is slightly different from actual semen, it still contains the exact same amount of sperms as regular semen.

This is why many people emphasize the fact that you must always wear a condom during intercourse at all times. Pulling out will not work due to pre-cum and there is no actual way for you to know when it will happen. Therefore, it is very possible to impregnate your partner if you were to be inside her without a condom.

Orgasm

This is the stage where you are going to orgasm. So, technically, you are not going to yet but you will. During this stage, you will feel your muscles tighten throughout the rest of your body and you will ejaculate.

There is a method that you can use to stop yourself from ejaculating, but we will discuss that in a later section. Anyhow, when you ejaculate, you will experience a euphoric feeling, especially at your lower abdominal muscles and that spasm will only last for about a fourth to a fifth of a second. After that, the feeling will subside after the outburst.

Note that it is possible to experience muscle aches on the next day.

Resolution

Once you've reached this stage, your erection will begin to die down as well as your breathing and heart rate. The good thing about the resolution stage is that it will help you during the second round.

Unfortunately, it will take up to an hour for you to reach another erection for the second stage. However, once the second round is reached, the orgasm stage will take a much longer time to appear because it will take time for all the sperm to accumulate again.

This is why masturbation can sometimes come in handy. It works the same way as going through regular intercourse. Best of all, for a man, masturbation is mostly an experimental stage to test your control of your body and to stop yourself form ejaculating when you don't want to.

Now that you've gotten a basic understanding of how your sexual levels are, it's time to move into the real purpose of this chapter: understand yourself.

In the next section, we will discuss your arousal patterns and, after that, we will talk about how to strengthen your PC muscles for better control of your body.

Your Arousal Patterns

Since every man is different, it also makes sense to say that your arousal patterns may be completely different than someone else's. However, the concept is still the same.

So in order for you to easily figure out your arousal patterns, you need to experiment, which means that you have to masturbate. You won't be able to experiment during sex because your mind will be too concentrated on your partner rather than your body.

If you have never masturbated before, now is the time. There are actually four steps to this process that you need to follow through, but it won't be anything difficult. Remember, this is an experiment that you are doing to figure yourself out, not to pleasure yourself. Don't be distracted, or else you will have to repeat the process from step one.

Remember to familiarize yourself with every level so you're able to easily pinpoint them during sex. By knowing how your body feels during each stage will allow you more control over it.

You should take as much time as you need, as there is no rush. If you feel that you weren't successful the first time then keep trying for the second or third time.

It doesn't matter how much you do it as long as you're able to improve after every session. Concentration is the key in this method and it is what you're aiming to do.

If you're able to familiarize yourself with the feelings you'll feel after each stage then you will have more control over your sexual responses during sex.

Stage 1

This would be twice as easy if there was no one else in the house but you. What you're going to need most is peace and quiet since you're going to need to heavily concentrate on yourself rather than the things around you.

It's best if you were to use the restroom when you're doing this since the restroom was designed for things like this. If you feel more comfortable in your bedroom, that is fine too.

Just make sure that you're willing to do the extra cleaning if anything were to go wrong. Once you've picked a set area, find a place to sit and sit up straight. You're not expected to maintain the perfect posture, but you also don't want to slouch.

Once you're in a good and comfortable position, it's time to stimulate yourself. You can use any method you want besides the use of porn and lube. Be creative and use your imagination. Men are visual creatures so it should be easy for you to do.

Stage 2

When you're finally erected, try to shift your mind to the feelings that you're having. Notice your breathing and heart rate. Start feeling whether your muscles are tightening or not. Try to take in every small detail that you can pinpoint from your body because the details that you notice as of now will be the details that will develop in the later stages.

Make sure to take it slowly. There is no rush in this process and it is possible for you to miss certain details when you're moving too quickly into the next step.

Stage 3

This is the part where you continue from stage two. Continue to stimulate yourself until you feel that you're about to reach your peaking point.

Even then, pay attention to how your body feels and how it changes. The more you're stimulated, the more your body will heat up and the faster your heart rate will be.

Your muscle will tighten even more the closer you are to your plateau stage because your body will be getting ready to ejaculate. Since the whole process is normally quick, you need to forcibly slow it down in order for you to completely feel the experience, as it should be felt.

Stage 4

This part is the last and most crucial part of the whole process. During this part, you will have to figure out when your ejaculation will occur.

Around this time, you no longer have the control over whether you want to ejaculate or not. You've already reached past the plateau of your erection and your orgasm will occur whether you like it or not.

However, keep that feeling intact. You want to know how you're feeling when you orgasm because it will also help you realize when your body will reach that point. After you start to remember the feeling of each stage, try to see if you're able to control the sensation that is transferring through your body.

You will not get it right the first time and it may even take much longer time than you anticipated. Nevertheless, you should keep trying until you've gotten the hang out it.

Normally, once you've reached stage four, you will not be able to control yourself from having the need to ejaculate. However, there is a last resort tactic that you can use in order to stop yourself from ejaculating at the last minute.

This technique is very advance and it will take a lot of practice to master. Nevertheless, in order to perform this technique in the first place, you will be required to strengthen up your PC muscles, something that we will discuss in the next section.

It's best to only try out this method after you've gotten yourself familiar with your arousal patterns. Not only will it smoothen out the process but it'll also make it easier to you to start.

You will need to start slowly in order to control your arousal patterns accurately. The faster you allow yourself to reach your peak, the faster you will ejaculate and the harder it will be for you to maintain control.

During the first step, you should focus on getting an erection and slowly maintaining it so it will not subside or burst.

The next step would require you use a part of your instincts. What you'll do is guestimate the time that you might ejaculate and stop yourself before you do.

In order to do this, you will need to flex your PC muscles extremely tight. If it helps, you may even flex your abs in the process. When you flex your PC muscles, make sure you hold it. Do not flex and let go within a few seconds. That will not do anything for you.

Since your breathing and heart rate may increase around this time, try not to take such deep breaths when you are flexing. If you do, it will become more difficult for you to continue flexing your muscles.

This part will be very important in determining whether you will cum or not.

As you are reaching the plateau stage of your erection, you will need to concentrate on balancing your arousal level so that you will not have an orgasm. You'll need to pay extra attention during this step even as you are having sex.

The point of this stage is to help lower your arousal as well as to keep you calm and relaxed while maintaining your excitement. You will, of course, feel minor spasms that feel as if you had orgasm the longer you try to maintain it. As long as you don't fully let go of your control completely, you will be fine. Remember, flexing is controlling.

Your PC Muscles

Now we'll talk about how to control your PC muscles. Your PC muscles are basically your pelvic muscles. It's what gives you endurance and power to control your arousal level, especially when you want to stop yourself from ejaculating.

There are a few PC muscle workouts that you can do to strengthen your PC muscles. However, we will only discuss the one that is most similar to what you have to do in the previous section.

Basically, it's a flexing workout. This is a short and simple workout that you can perform anywhere you want because it does not require any movement from the any other parts of your body.

So what you do when you start is to flex your PC muscles and hold the position for up to three seconds. Not that bad right? Once the three seconds have passed, release your muscles and relax for up to three seconds.

You should do about 20 sets of these each for up to three times a day. Remember to take deep breaths as you flex and release. Proper breathing also leads to a proper workout with proper results. If possible, do not do this exercise with a full erection, especially when you first start off.

Chapter 3 - Premature Ejaculation

Now that you know the basics of your sexual levels and how to control them, it's about time that we talk about premature ejaculations.

Although the issue might not be heard of very often, it's very big problem for men and their sex lives. Of course, how many men do you know that would easily accept and admit the fact that they go through premature ejaculations?

It would mostly be from zero to none. It's a sexual dysfunction that many, if not all, men is afraid of experiencing.

Since men want to be considered good, if not great, in bed, having to deal with premature ejaculation will only deteriorate their pride and confidence as a man. Unfortunately, most men do suffer from premature ejaculation whether they admit it or not.

For most people, the issue isn't as big of a deal for them as others. Each reaction is based on the current circumstances that a man is faced with at the moment and, for many, it's a huge dilemma.

Although some men do not make such a big deal out of it for themselves, they still have their partner as a reason. For women who are with men that go through premature ejaculations, it can be a huge deal for her, especially if she wants to get pregnant.

Sadly, premature ejaculation can happen even before the actual intercourse, which will completely frustrate the woman that has to deal with it.

For those of you that are suffering the heavy side of premature ejaculation, it's best if you were to treat it as soon as possible. Even if your partner tells you that she doesn't mind now, she will in the long run.

Before we can move into the solution of getting rid of premature ejaculation, we have to first understand how it works and how it develops.

In the first section we'll talk more about how premature ejaculation works and the causes of it. Afterwards, we'll talk about the possible ways to cure premature ejaculations. In addition, we'll also mention some myths about premature ejaculations that you might find interested in knowing.

Functions and Causes

Premature ejaculation is simply the process of ejaculating too soon. Normally, an average healthy man can last about 2-6 minutes in bed before ejaculating. However, those who suffer from premature ejaculations can only last about thirty seconds to one minute.

If they're lucky then maybe two minutes. Either way, the time of pleasure is cut off during sex and you have no control over it. Just so you know, premature ejaculation isn't a disease. It is an issue and it is not something that you can take medication for and hope that it'll go away.

Despite the fact that it takes a man a maximum of six minutes to ejaculate still doesn't necessarily cut it for a woman. Unlike men, women can take up to fifteen minutes to achieve a full out orgasm, which sucks because men usually don't know what to do after they're done before their partner is.

Fortunately, it is possible to shorten her time if you know what to do, but that will be details covered in another chapter.

Nevertheless, the great aspect about a woman is the fact that they don't need to be thrusts into to achieve an orgasm. There are other methods out there that don't require you to be in her for her to gain pleasure.

The tricky part about premature ejaculation is the fact that it can happen to anyone at any time. In addition, it's also not steady.

For a man who did not have sex for a certain amount of time, he will most likely go through premature ejaculation during his first intercourse.

Now, that won't be a problem unless if it continues for every intercourse that he has. If that were to happen then he would need to be immediately treated.

You never want to get too comfortable with having premature ejaculation even if you are not currently dating. It's not something that you want to have to deal with in the long run.

There are a few reasons as to why men will suffer through premature ejaculation. Some of which will include genetics, stress and anxiety, an unhealthy lifestyle, poor masturbation methods, and wrong posturing.

Genetics

This reason has nothing to do with your actions. You are simply one of the many that were born with this issue at hand. It is very rare for a man to last even six minutes during an intercourse so you can guess how low of a percentage of the male population that is.

Because we are mammals, it is only right that we cannot last a long time in bed. The way Mother Nature has set it out for us is that we could reproduce as quickly as possible.

That was the point of intercourse back then: to enter, ejaculate, and impregnate your partner. Nowadays, sex has a deeper meaning into it.

Unfortunately, long lasting pleasure is not something that life has laid out for us yet.

Stress and Anxiety

Usually, when people do say that attitude is important, it's always best to listen to them. It doesn't matter who says it because it's true.

Your attitude does reflect a lot on your behavior and your mentality. Having a positive mentality is actually beneficial for your health. So what does that mean?

It means that if you're suffering through stress and anxiety then that is probably a likely reason as to why you suffer through premature ejaculation. Although it may take a while for you to realize how stressed out you are at the moment, your body will make you realize it in the long run.

When you prepare for sex, you want to be free of any thoughts that you have at the moment. It doesn't matter if it's important because that should've been finished and taken care of before you decided that it was pleasure time.

Many men who worry too much about ejaculating too soon in bed will end up ejaculating too soon in bed because the constant fear is on their mind. They are focusing too much on their possible mistake rather than the pleasure that they can receive.

If you are in a heated moment, don't let your stress and fear ruin it for you.

An Unhealthy Lifestyle

Nowadays, being unhealthy is like a trend. Practically more than half of the U.S. population is considered unhealthy, or even close to it. You might think that being unhealthy is all right as long as you don't cross a certain point in your weight, but once you've been deemed unhealthy then you are unhealthy.

In fact, being unhealthy does not mean that you are too overweight or too underweight. Your weight is only a part of your health as there are other factors that decide it for you.

Of course, your food intake is important too since it's going into your stomach. You should be careful as to what type of food you're consuming on a daily basis. It's fine to have sugar as long as it's not in huge doses, or it's taken every single day.

High calorie food is also bad for you and can damage your blood circulation system. Just so you know, premature ejaculation can also happen from poor blood flow. If you do end up eating unhealthy foods for one day, do make the effort to exercise it off on that same day, if not the next day.

By prolonging the need to exercise, you're only going to make your body feel a lot worse than before.

Poor Masturbation Methods

Yea, it sounds weird but it's possible if you think about it. Masturbating is like having sex minus the penetration. It's like air sex basically, and you're doing it alone.

Anyways, the way you masturbate can affect your sex life, and it is possible to suffer through premature ejaculation in the long run because of it.

When you masturbate, you're not just trying to reach an orgasm as quickly as you can. By masturbating too quickly all the time, you run the risk of suffering through premature ejaculation during actual sex.

What's worse is that the issue is more prone to young men who do this early on in their lifetime. Of course, that doesn't mean that older men won't run the same risk as the younger ones.

The Wrong Posturing

Sometimes, your posture during sex can also be the reason why you go through premature ejaculation. There's a reason why most people tend to switch positions every once in a while.

If you haven't done so, it's best if you start trying. Even though positions during sex might not seem like a big deal, each position can give a certain amount of pleasure to it.

In addition, each position can also cause different side effects after you're done. You don't have to try every sex position known to man. It's just good to know a small variety in case if one doesn't work out for you.

How to Cure Yourself

The issue with premature ejaculation is the fact that men tend to ignore it rather than seek help for it.

Fortunately, it is a treatable dysfunction; however, because so many men tend to keep it to themselves, the problem becomes impossible to fix. Sorry to disappoint you, but your premature ejaculation issues aren't going to fix itself.

Although it may be embarrassing to talk about, it's the first step that you have to take in order to find a cure. As previously mentioned, there is a high risk of suffering through premature ejaculation when you tend to finish masturbating too quickly.

It's simply something that your body has gotten used to from your own past habits. So now, all you have to do, is to reverse those old habits.

In this section, we are going to talk about how to permanently cure you from premature ejaculation. So what does that mean? It means that the methods that we will talk about will not include any expensive medication.

Nowadays, since most men are too shy to admit to their faults, top companies and commercial firms have taken advantage of that. The whole deal with long lasting pills, specialized condoms, and even sprays have been mass-produced to attract men looking for a solution to their problems.

However, those solutions are not permanent. Sure, it may work for a while, but it's also going to cost you a lot of money in the long run. Also, what seems more embarrassing in to your end?

The fact that you have to rely on products to help you last longer or the fact that you can't last longer, period.

When you want to find a cure of premature ejaculation, you're looking for a cure that helps solve your issue and do no harm to your sexual experience.

Fortunately, the best cure is the most natural cure, which means that it's about time you start adopting some training programs that will help your body withstand mental and physical stimulation.

We'll go over those natural exercises near the end of the book since it'll be easier for you to find it if you want to go back and review.

Premature Ejaculation Myths

This section will quickly cover the myths and lies about premature ejaculation. Although the topic may not be as important as the rest of the book, it's still useful information that you should consider.

Not only that, knowing the truth about these myths will indeed help you boost up your confidence for the next time you decide to have sex as well as help you avoid certain methods during sex.

Lack of Sexual Experience

In a sense, this myth is true; however, it's true to a certain extent. There is a high chance of men experiencing premature ejaculation during their first intercourse.

That is completely normal since it is a new experience for them. Just like how some women will start off bad at sex, men can too. It goes for any physical intimacy that any couples have.

In addition, premature ejaculation can also happen for those who have barely resumed sex after a long hiatus.

There is also nothing wrong with that because their body simply needs to readjust to the sensation again.

Unfortunately, if you're suffering through premature ejaculation and you have had experience with sex, it means that you are seriously suffering from premature ejaculation.

Don't diminish your own sexual experience if you've got plenty. It doesn't mean that you're bad in bed, but simply because you come too soon.

Experience really has little to do with premature ejaculation than your body itself. Also, by believing that you are bad in bed, your anxiety will grow and it will affect your actual performance in bed, causing you to become what you feared becoming.

Porn Actors Have it Easy

On the contrary, they don't. Porn actors are forced to be good in bed. That's their job and that's what they are paid to do.

Now it may sound easy but they are expected to last a little longer than what the average man can do, which is a lot.

Besides, most porn actors have a high chance of experiencing what you have multiple times in the industry. Even if they are good, they are not perfect. It won't be a surprise if they will suffer through premature ejaculation once in a while.

It's all thanks to their training that they are able to last that long so don't feel bad if you're unable to last as long as they are able to.

You Have Issues

If you suffer through premature ejaculation, there is nothing wrong with you. If someone is making you think that way then they are probably lucky enough to not experience it yet or they are being insensitive and trying to drag you down.

Yet, never fear, for they will eventually. As mentioned before, premature ejaculation is not a physical dysfunction. It just means that you cannot last in bed as long as another man.

Men are not expected to last in bed for a long time and women know that. However, they do expect for you to know your way around. Basically, if you can last over a minute before ejaculating, all you have to do is brush up your technique in order to last for as long as you want.

Distractions

If any advice magazine or catalog has ever told you that being distracted helps, it really doesn't. In the end, it's all about how you want to go with it.

Sure, by distracting yourself, you may be able to slow down your ejaculation time. However, it means that you won't be able to experience the same sexual pleasure that you can be experiencing if you paid attention to what you were doing.

Unless if you are having sex just to get it over with, forcibly distracting yourself is not the way to go.

It's Not the End

Although premature ejaculation can heavily damage your self-esteem during sex, keep in mind that it's not really all that bad.

Sure, you've reached your peak before your partner did, but she obviously knows that you can't help it. Either way, just because you came before your partner doesn't mean that you still can't make her come.

Sex isn't just about the penetrating and thrusting. Sex is also a way for you and your partner to be sexually intimate with each other.

It takes the average man about 30 minutes to an hour before he is able to get another erection. At the same time, it takes a woman a maximum of 15 minutes before she is able to orgasm.

The twist is the fact that it takes more effort for men to orgasm in the second round while it takes less to zero effort for women to orgasm in the second round.

Basically, if you are able to distract your partner and give her an orgasm before you recover for the second round of sex, you are still good to go.

Your partner is not going to care that much if you come before her. In fact, she'll be amazed if you don't. However, that doesn't mean that she expects less from you. The only thing that your woman will expect from you during sex is what you do to give her an orgasm.

Do not be immediately discouraged if things don't go the way you planned it to. Act quickly and use other methods that you know or have learned.

Penetration isn't the only thing that will arouse her. Once you've gain more experience in lovemaking, you'll realize that your hands and tongues will be the best parts of your body in bed.

Besides, a woman will naturally be turned on if you remain confident the whole time during sex.

Chapter 4 - Being Healthy and Safe

In the previous section, we mentioned about getting into exercises. For now, we'll talk about how to stay fit in order to perform those exercises.

When you start any type of exercise, you don't immediately start with the toughest workout. You start easy as your body slowly build up stamina for the next type of workout.

Then, slowly and slowly, you start to be able to perform more advanced workouts. At the same time, however, you must also pay close attention to your health. Exercising to stay healthy doesn't do much to your health if you don't eat healthy.

We also mentioned before that your premature ejaculation issues could be from the cause of an unhealthy lifestyle. So your food consumption is also something that you have to take note of if you want a successful sex life.

In this chapter we'll be taking a quick glance at the type of nutrients you should eat on a daily basis and what you should avoid. Afterwards, we'll move towards some safety tips that you should know about your exercise workout so you can get started as soon as possible.

Necessary Nutrients

Water. The only drink you should ever consume on a daily basis is water. Water is especially important for your health. You can last days without food but you can't last one day without water.

That is a fact. It is recommended that you drink about 3-4 bottles of water per day in order to obtain the proper amount of nutrients that you need.

However, you don't want to consume five or more bottles. Although water may be good for you, you should only drink a moderate amount.

Drinking too much water can damage your health. That means that you should also cut down on your sugar intake. Most sodas and manufactured drinks have plenty of sugar in it.

Even if the brand specifically states diet, it's still enough sugar for you to want more. If you're tired of drinking water then tea should be your second option. Only drink carbonated drinks once in a while, and not too much at once.

Eating food with enough vitamins will also help improve your health. That means eating more vegetables and fruits on a daily basis.

So get rid of your daily habit of consuming too much junk food in one day, or eating them everyday. That doesn't mean that you have to completely rid yourself of junk food all together.

What you want to do is to cut the portion down and only eat them every once in a while. They are unhealthy for a reason. Who knows, after a while, you might even see a change in your overall penis size.

Safety Tips

Please note that in order to obtain the best results, you need to follow up with the exercise plan as accurately as possible. If you end up skipping a step or mess up, there is a possible chance where you can injure yourself.

During your first time, move slowly and carefully. Once you're used the workout, you can move in the pace that you want. Always make sure to do the warm-up exercises required before heading off to the actual work out.

Warm-up exercises are there for a reason. It's the same with regular exercises. You have to stretch your body before starting on any intense exercises so you don't run the risk of damaging your tendons.

Do note that you should consult with a doctor to see if there's anything wrong with you in the first place. There may be some cases where it might not be premature ejaculation but an actual dysfunction.

Since you'll need to use lubricant throughout the workout, there might be some products that your skin is allergic to.

Either way, consult with a doctor and ask him as much questions as possible before starting on anything. If, during any time in the workout, you start to experience some issues with your penis, make sure that you go see a doctor immediately since they will know what to do.

Lubricant

Since you'll be starting on your penis enhancement exercises soon, you'll need to choose a proper lubricant in order to obtain the best result without inflicting any damage to yourself.

This is especially important because it is possible to obtain an infection if you aren't careful enough. Do not buy some cheap lubricant because you don't want to waste money.

Any product that has to do with your body should be considered carefully no matter how expensive it is. If you aren't careful, it is possible that you can end up with skin irritation throughout the duration of the exercise and all your efforts may become fruitless.

So what kind of lubricant you should take into consideration you ask? For one thing, you want to buy a lubricant that can last for a whole session throughout the exercise that you do.

Having to constantly reapply lubricant during a workout session can also lower the efficiency rate of your workout. With that in mind, you need to pay extra attention when choosing what kind of lube that you're buying.

If you're not the type to read every detail in a product then now is about time. You need to note the brand, packaging, and quality of the lubricant that you're going to buy.

If you aren't sure then do some extra research before heading off to the store and buying some. It'll probably save you a lot of time. If the lubricant that you're aiming for is only available online, try seeing how fast it'll take for the product to reach you. After all, you do want to start as soon as possible.

Chapter 5 - Exercises

Now that we've finally moved onto the exercise portion of the book, there will be some exercise workouts that you will be able to use.

Although there is already some exercises spread throughout the book, these will be the main ones that you will work it in order to improve your penis size.

Note that it does not contain every single work out that is known to man. If you want additional workouts that are not included in this book, you can always research them online.

As this was mentioned in the previous chapter, you should note that it is possible to sustain injuries if you are not performing these workout sessions properly.

It is crucial that you follow the instructions given to the best of your abilities. In addition, it is best to get yourself treated and tested by a doctor before starting. For all you know, you might be experiencing another problem that is similar to what you thought it was.

Throughout each exercise, if you feel that there might be something wrong with you or if you're developing a rash or any problems that does not seem normal, it is best if you were to consult with a doctor immediately.

Do not let it sit and wait for it to die out. If you become sore or experience blisters, stop doing the exercises until it heals. Consult to your doctor for any type of doubts you have during the whole process. They are there to help you.

Remember, these exercises will not give you overnight results. They will take time, effort, and dedication. You are free to do these exercises any time you want during the day.

However, in order to experience the best results, you must be consistent with your efforts. Even if it will take a long time, there will be results. As you perform these exercises on a consistent basis, you move one step closer to your goals.

Nevertheless, you should not do these exercises every day. After each exercise, you must allow your penis to heal for at least two days before continuing again. Sure, the wait time might slow you down but, in reality, it will help.

Within this chapter we will go over warm-ups that you will need to do before each exercise, the basic exercises that you can do, and how to cool down after each workout.

Warm-Ups

Every type of exercise needs a certain set of warm-ups, whether it's stretching, taking a light jog, or breathing warm-ups, you need them in order to prepare your body for the actual workout.

Although warm-ups are simple to do, they can affect the whole performance of your actual workout if you do not perform them properly. Therefore, make sure that you take each warm-up exercise seriously as if it was a real one.

Besides, the warm-ups for penis enhancement is fairly easy to accomplish and will take little effort to finish.

A Warm Shower

Whether you choose to shower or bath all depends on your preferences. Either way, you are giving heat to your penis. The reason why this is necessary is because the warm water will help loosen up the tissues within that area so it will be easier for you perform more advance work-outs.

Hot Wraps

If you don't want to take a shower or a bath then grab a small towel, rinse it through warm water, and wrap it around your penis. Make sure that the towel is warm all around and that it is not too wet or too dry.

Leave the warm towel around your penis for about two minutes before redoing the steps again for a second time. Repeat this process about three times.

In the end, this process can take up to about 8 minutes, which is also the same amount of time it can take you to shower or bathe.

Passing Your Limits

This exercise will mainly focus on extending your arousal time without ejaculating. Since men can only last for a maximum of six minutes before ejaculation, they have a disadvantage during sex.

However, for this exercise, we will work on extending your six minutes into fifteen, which is the same amount of time a woman will take to orgasm.

When starting, make sure that you are able to give yourself an erection without the help of porn, lube, and any other methods besides your hands. Move yourself towards the sixth level on your arousal scale and stop.

Make sure that your erection is still up and ready even if you were to relax your muscles. Wait until your level drops down to four before starting again. Repeat this step about five times before moving on.

Now, repeat the first step again but bring your level up to eight and then back down to six. Repeat the process another five times before moving on.

Keep up this pattern until you've reached your maximum level. It is fine if you cannot do it the first time since this method will take some time to master.

The Jelqing Technique

The Jelqing technique is actually a very old technique that is commonly used for penis enhancement. What these exercises do is make your penis larger by allowing more blood space.

Best of all, the results are permanent and it will enlarge both the flaccid and erect state. However, this technique should not be practiced everyday. It is best if you were to keep it to a maximum of five days a week in order to allow your penis to rest.

This is the simplest technique for the Jelqing. Basically, you start by applying lubricant to your flaccid penis from the hilt to the head.

By using only the thumb and forefinger, start to stretch your penis downward and slightly outward. When you do this, it's best to be gentle but firm at the same time.

You don't want to hurt yourself but you want to apply some sort of force to keep the position steady. Once you've gotten the position aligned, start milking yourself. If you've never seen anyone milk a cow then you basically hold your penis and start switching hands while stretching your penis downward and outward. Repeat this step 100 times before stopping.

After a week or so, start moving that 100 times to 200 times. The tricky part about this technique is that your penis will become red and might swell up. However, that is perfectly normal because it means that more blood is traveling into your penis.

The Natural Technique

This technique can be found online if you were to search for it. It is a basic two step technique that will help stretch the length of your overall penis. This is a technique that you will have to do when you're flaccid. It will not work if you have an erection so do not bother.

Basically, you have to take one hand and firmly grip around the tip of your penis. Do not grip hard enough so that you start to cut off any blood circulation. That is not what we are trying to do.

Once you've gotten your grip perfected, start pulling your penis out in front of you until you start to feel a good and painless stretch in your penis.

Make sure that you're able to hold that position for up to thirty seconds before letting yourself rest. If you mess up then redo the process. Continue this technique for about 10-15 minutes before you let yourself take a 20-minute break.

Cooling Down

After finish your workout of the day, you need to cool your penis down because it is important that you allow it to recover. It's like taking a mile-jog.

Once you're done running, it's recommended that you walk for another lap to cool your body down before sitting down and relaxing.

Your penis requires the same method. In addition, cooling down help stop your penis from sustaining any injuries that you could have possibly cause during the exercise.

In order to cool your penis down, you need to massage it for about three minutes max. Make sure that you are no longer in your erect stage but your flaccid stage. Once you're done with the massage, repeat the same process as you would for the warm-up section by either doing the hot wraps or taking a warm shower.

Chapter 6 - Improving Your Skills

This is going to be a short and quick session about how to improve your skills in bed. Remember, women may take up to fifteen minutes to reach their first orgasm and men can only last up to six minutes before theirs.

However, women don't necessarily enjoy the idea of you coming before she does. So in this chapter, we'll be focusing on what you can do to help your partner reach her orgasm before you do.

Intercourse isn't the only technique that you can do to give your partner an orgasm. Luckily, within those fifteen minutes of sex, there are plenty of other techniques that you can do to make her come. As long as she's feeling the sensation then her body will automatically respond to you.

Making Sure Your Partner is Relaxed

Before you head off into any type of sexual intercourse, you want to make sure that your partner is relaxed and calm.

If you try to penetrate her when her body is not relaxed, you can potentially harm her no matter lightly you're thrusting into her.

Also, if she is feeling uncomfortable during the intercourse, there is a high chance that she will not be turned on for anything that you do and that it will take a much longer time for her to achieve orgasm.

If you're having trouble moving past this stage no matter what you do, it's probably the fact that it has something to do with your surroundings. The ambience around the room is important for a woman when you want to make love to her.

However, they are not expecting anything extravagant. All they want to see is a clean and fresh smelling room. If you want to add in the extra fancy scented candles and soft music then by all means, go for it.

Just remember, a woman takes note of what you will do even if it is a slight insignificant thing.

The Practice Round

Although practice rounds may be odd and weird before the actual thing, it does help. If you haven't realized it yet, it takes a longer time for a man to orgasm a second time compared to the first.

Unfortunately, it also takes off some pleasure into sex during the second round. You can think of it as an exchange, basically. If you don't really have much of a care into the issue then this method would be good for you.

Basically, what you should do is to masturbate about an hour before the actual intercourse. The way this work is that you will be cleansing your system and it'll take another hour for your body to reproduce the amount of sperm that you wasted when you masturbate.

The best part is the fact that your partner will not know unless if you make it too obvious, of course. So if you want an easy way to last a little longer in bed, this will be a good method to do.

If you don't want to masturbate then there's always the option of going for the second round with your partner.

So instead of a solo practice round, do both with your partner. Besides, if she didn't feel much pleasure in the first round, she might not mind going for another one as long as you can prove yourself for the second round.

Using a Condom

Every man should wear a condom during intercourse unless if the purpose is to impregnate your partner. Although the rubber on the condom won't give you as much pleasure as skin-to-skin contact, it provides protection for both you and your partner.

If you don't like wearing one then it's time to learn. There are plenty of brands out there so you have a wide variety of choosing the one that matches your preferences the most.

Also, a condom can really help you last longer during intercourse. Basically, what a condom can do is restrict your blood flow due to the tightness if gives you when you're wearing it.

Try to experiment with different brands and types of condoms until you find one that you really love using.

Distractions

We mentioned before in the previous chapter(s) about how you should not distract yourself during intercourse. However, that doesn't mean that the rule also applies to your partner.

In fact, during intercourse, you want to distract her. She doesn't care about what you do as long as she's receiving the pleasure that she wants.

Sex isn't just about penetration. Play with her for a bit and let her take control every once in a while. It's a lot easier for you to come first when you're always in control.

By letting your partner have her control over you, you have the time to relax for a bit and let her do the work. Then, once you start feeling yourself coming, stop your partner and distract her with some playful tactics until your body calms down again.

The point is, use every method you know that doesn't just include penetration. There are also kissing, fingering, and even massaging. Every woman enjoys a good massage so if you're good with your hands, that's a plus.

Remember, every woman likes to be in control at a certain point during sex. If you can let her do what she wants, and easily reclaim your control over her without her realizing it then sex will be a whole lot easier for you from now on.

Positioning

Position is indeed important for a great sex experience. There are a lot of sex positions out there, but too little time to test out every one of them.

However, there is enough time for at least two positions during intercourse if you know how to plan out your timings properly. From there on, you can always try out new positions every time you and your partner have sex to see which positions matches you the best.

Sure enough, there are some sex positions out there that will give you more control over your body than others. The basic sex position that most couples do is the missionary, which indefinitely gives you less control over your own body due to the stress over your muscles.

A few great positions that you should keep in mind is the basic cowgirl and spoon. The cowgirl is when your partner is on top of you.

This position is perfect for you to use when you want to control your ejaculation time simply because you aren't doing any work into the thrusting.

By lying on your back, you're allowing your partner to do the work while you're relaxing. The spoon, on the other hand, is when both you and your partner are laying on your sides, and her back is facing towards you as you penetrate her.

This position gives you the power to control how your thrusts are and it'll also let your partner feel the intimacy between the both of you.

Her Sensitive Areas

Women have a few sensitive areas that can easily arouse them during sex. In normal situations, those areas won't do much but it's a different story when you're in bed with her.

Once you're able to pinpoint what these areas are, learn to work around it. When you're in bed with her, let her believe that she knows what you're going to do.

Make your next move obvious, but unexpected. Show her that you're aiming for a certain spot and quickly move on to another.

That unexpected gesture will get her going even more because she won't be prepared for it. Also, don't immediately head off to those sensitive spots of hers.

Play around it and wait awhile before attacking it. Be creative during sex because creativity is what's going to help you make her come.

The Ears

Ears are sensitive, but it won't turn your partner on if you're not touching the right spot. During sex, take a chance at nibbling her earlobes, or you can even lick around her ears if it's easier for you.

Because she's already in the mood, triggering her sensitive area will make it a whole lot easier to get her aroused.

Also, if you're confident of your voice then try whispering to her. Women especially love it when a man whispers in her ears during sex. If you know that she loves your voice then you've already gained a good position.

The Spine

If you've never brushed your fingers against your partner's spine during sex, it's bout time you do. However, there's a trick to it.

Even if your partner is not ticklish, she can still feel a little tingle when you brush your fingers against her spine. You just have to make sure that you're doing it slowly and gently. Make sure that you're doing it near the end of her spine and not the top or the middle.

This will work perfectly when she's on top of you or has her back towards you. You'll know you've hit the right spot when she gives a little twitch to her body the moment you brush your hands on her.

Just remember that it only work if you do it once in a while during sex. If you constantly do it in succession then she'll probably be squirming all over you and it's going to turn her off.

The Neck

The neck is a tricky area simply because the throat is there too. If you're applying too much pressure to her neck, you can end up making her feel as if she's being chocked by you.

Thus, you'll be turning her off before you even have the chance to make a comeback. However, if you're applying the right amount of pressure, it'll make her feel great.

If your woman is especially ticklish around the neck area then you have to be a little more careful so she doesn't start having an outburst of laughter while you're trying to turn her on.

Nevertheless, if you ever get the chance then aim for the back of her neck where the spine starts. Most women are extra sensitive around that part. Although it might not all be in the same area, trying moving around to find the spot where she is extra sensitive at.

Oral Sex

Oral sex is very popular among couples in bed simply because it is the easiest besides penetration. If you are fine with performing oral sex on your partner then be sure to use that to your advantage.

In fact, most women prefer oral sex over penetrative sex simply because it's a lot more satisfying for them. Not to mention that there's no actual movement on their part. The thing with women is the fact that they can have multiple orgasms during one session.

Usually, their first orgasms are a lot more difficult to bring out compare to any succeeding orgasms. Thus, if you can make her orgasm using oral sex before the actual intercourse, you'll have a lot more easier time making her feel great in bed. In addition, as an added bonus, it'll also boost up your confidence in bed.

The reason why oral sex can provide much more pleasure than penetrative sex is because there's more freedom involved. During penetrative sex, the only movement that a woman can really feel is your thrusting.

Thus, your body is only moving in and out of her body. However, for oral sex, your tongue is free to move anywhere around her clitoris.

Now, although oral sex may seem easy to accomplish, there is a difficult part to it. For the first few sessions, women will expect a man to be bad at it.

Unless if she knows that you have performed oral sex before, she will not expect much from you during your first time with her. Regardless of that, there is no fixed way to stimulate her using oral sex, meaning that you are free to do what you please.

There is no fixed method as everyone does it differently. Yet, because of that, it gives you space to be creative. If you're the type that moves by instincts, this should be a fun way for you to arouse your partner.

A really good method you can use if you're stuck is to form letters. Start tracing the ABCs with your tongue on her clitoris and give variations to each movement. Basically, when you are giving her oral sex, try to soften up your tongue for the most part.

However, there are times when you want to add pressure to her clitoris using your tongue. It'll give you a little variation to work with and she won't be feeling the same sensitivity all of the time.

What you should keep in mind when giving your partner oral sex is to be careful of how she reacts. Before you start digging yourself deep into her, pay attention to her reactions first.

Chances are, if she isn't feeling aroused then that means that she's feeling uncomfortable. Therefore, that's your number one sign to stop what you're doing and try something else.

It's Not About You

Really, it's not. When you are having sex with your partner, you have to focus more on her than yourself.

It's not going to be about what kind of pleasure you feel but about what kind of pleasure that she'll feel.

The reason why is because once a man is aroused, he's going to stay aroused until he ejaculates within six minutes. However, when a woman is aroused, she's got a whole fifteen minutes to feel some intense pleasure.

Besides, when you're having sex, you're mostly thinking about how to make your partner feel good. It's very easy, but difficult to do.

During sex, your partner needs to be in your mind all of the time. You have to notice all her slight movements, gestures, and reactions. Those are your clues to figuring how she's feeling during sex.

Do not expect her to tell you how she's feeling. Not many women will bother telling you when she's turned on and there is no way in hell is she going to direct your movements for you.

There's a thick line between a woman taking charge during sex and when she has to tell you what to do during sex. You want the first one and not the other.

Do realize that not every single sex tip you pick is going to work. Every woman is different so there is a possible chance that your partner may desire the complete opposite of what other women wants.

So if you're planning to ask your female friends about what woman wants in bed, she's not going to be much help if they are completely different people.

The Aftermath

After the intense sex that both you and your partner just went through, try to not let yourself fall asleep so easily.

Even if your partner had fallen asleep before you have, stay up for a little more anyways. The reason why is so you can cuddle her.

Women are emotional creatures so it's a bonus for you if you let her know how much you care through physical contact.

Even if she might not feel it during her sleep, she will when she wakes up. The best part is that you don't even have to give her a bear hug or anything of the sort. Just simply wrap your arms around her body and stay by her side for the night.

Conclusion

From what you've learned up until now, take it in and do it. The exercises included within this book will not give you results over night. They will take weeks and even months until you've reached the results that you want.

Take note of the skills mentioned in this book. Remember it, keep it in your head, and visualize it.

Although you won't be perfect immediately, as long as you have the idea in mind then it will flow naturally when you make love with your partner.

By reading this book, you've already made the first step towards a better sex life with your partner. You've already started taking the first step so why not advance to the second step as soon as you can.

Take a few minutes per day to perform the exercises listed in this book and try out the different techniques provided for you whenever you do it.

There is nothing for you to fear since the worst that can happen is the fact that your partner is dissatisfied.

However, that gives you even more of a reason to try harder the next time. Don't let one or two sessions drag you down, and don't let a your premature ejaculation take control of your confidence. Remember, sex is not end until you decide that it will end.

Don't tear yourself up because you're not getting the results you want. Good things come to those who wait, and better things happen for those who put in the effort for it.

Give it time and you will start seeing the results you want. As long as you maintain your confidence, brush up on your techniques, and work on your penis enhancement sessions, your results will come.

Soon enough, you'll realize that your sex life will be completely different from how it was before.

www.ingramcontent.com/pod-product-compliance
Lightning Source LLC
Chambersburg PA
CBHW020355290526
45785CB00005B/2303